SWALLOWING DISORDERS

A Guide To Managing Dysphagia
In The Elderly

By

S. G. Garbin

* * * * *

PUBLISHED BY:
S.G. Garbin

DEDICATION

To caregivers everywhere.
You make all the difference.

TABLE OF CONTENTS

INTRODUCTION

If you are sitting down to a delicious meal right now, you are doing something that millions of people, affected by a swallowing disorder, are unable to do. Many elderly or neurologically impaired individuals can no longer enjoy a traditional holiday meal or even drink a glass of water without fear of choking or developing a lung infection.

Dysphagia, a technical term for a swallowing disorder, occurs in both adult and pediatric populations, however, the focus of this guide is identifying the challenges associated with caring for elderly people afflicted with dysphagia. This book is designed with you, the caregiver, in mind. It offers an overview of the changes in chewing and swallowing that often occur as people age or in the presence of serious neurological or cognitive diseases such as Alzheimer's or stroke. This book is a tool to help you and your loved one or those in your care compensate for the loss of chewing and swallowing abilities.

I hope you find it helpful and I would love to receive feedback from readers. Please check the back of the book under the heading *Author* if you would like to connect with me on a variety of social media sites.

CHAPTER 1

THE PROCESS OF SWALLOWING-NORMAL AND IMPAIRED

Eating is simple, right? You take a bite of food, chew it and swallow it. It sure seems that way until something happens to make chewing and swallowing a chore. Something that we take for granted hundreds of times (bites and sips) per day can run the gamut from nuisance to down right scary when our ability to do it goes awry.

The technical term for problems with chewing or swallowing is Dysphagia (dis-fay-gee-uh or sometimes pronounced dis-fah-juh). If the problem is in the mouth, the diagnosis is "oral dysphagia." If it is primarily a problem with clearing foods at the level of the throat (Pharynx), it is called "pharyngeal dysphagia." It is possible to have a combination of problems, particularly if the patient (spouse or father—these terms will be used interchangeably) has suffered a stroke or has other neurological problems.

To better understand what can go wrong with swallowing, let's take a look at the normal process first.

Anatomy and Function

Believe it or not, the tongue plays as vital a role in swallowing as it does in forming words for speech. The tongue and other muscles in our mouth and throat are responsible for our ability to speak and use our voices, however they are also used for chewing and swallowing function.

During typical speech production, the tongue must be able to make complicated movements to clearly produce (articulate) each individual sound. If you combine that with the complexity of adding multiple sounds together to form words and then string those words together to create phrases and sentences, it is pretty obvious that speech is a complicated process. Any disruption in the strength, coordination or range of motion of this muscle group can affect both speech and swallowing.

Coordinating our breathing is also a factor in speaking and safely swallowing foods. Dysfunction occurs when an individual is weak all over or has reduced lung capacity. Signs that he is having trouble may start with his speech. He may have an increasingly soft voice or may not be loud enough. He may become "winded" if he tries to talk a great deal. This is commonly observed in individuals with COPD (Chronic Obstructive Pulmonary Disease) who have a history of smoking or nonsmoking related lung problems. A stroke or diagnosis of a disease such as Parkinson's disease may result in significant weakness in these muscles as well as the muscles used in breathing.

Dysarthria, a clinical term for such weakness and can affect any muscle tissue including the mouth, throat and abdominal muscles. It makes sense, that, if speech is slurred, soft, or hypernasal speech, the muscles are weak and likely not well coordinated. If he uses an oxygen tank because he has reduced lung capacity, this will affect how loud his speech is and how long he is able to talk.

Conclusion: If he has trouble talking and coordinating his breathing, he may have trouble chewing and swallowing.

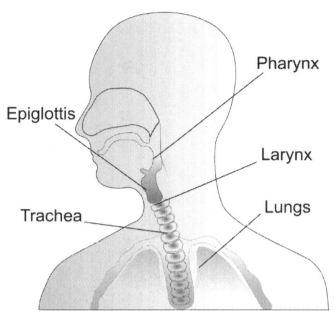

Description: English: Recreation of Diagram of the Human Throat.*

ORAL/ORAL PREPARATORY PHASE (CHEWING)

The structures involved: Tongue, lips, jaw, cheeks/chewing muscles, soft palate, hard palate.

SUMMARY OF STAGES

- A bite of food or a sip of liquid is taken.
- Foods are broken down and mixed with saliva.
- A soft ball of chewed food (bolus) is formed and trapped between the tongue and the hard palate
- The soft palate lifts to seal the nasal cavity as the tongue pushes the bolus toward the throat (pharynx) for swallowing.
- The bolus is swallowed.

That sounds pretty easy, doesn't it? In reality, the oral phase of swallowing is more complex than most people realize. Impairment of this phase may lead to signs and symptoms of choking or aspiration (foods and liquids entering the lungs). While choking can lead to death, chronic aspiration can lead to pneumonia or chronic upper respiratory illness over time, which can also be fatal if not caught and treated by a physician. Chewing just got a whole lot more complicated, didn't it?

Let's take a further look at the difference between a normal and impaired chewing (oral preparatory phase).

NORMAL CHEWING

During the oral preparatory phase, foods are mixed with saliva and broken down by the teeth. The tongue sweeps and collects foods into a soft ball (bolus), and channels chewed foods to the opening of the throat for swallowing. The result is a bolus (ball) of masticated food that can then be swallowed. The soft palate (velum) lifts and seals off the nasal cavity during the process of swallowing. The tongue creates a channel that transports thin liquids to the correct place for swallowing. Tongue impairment may lead to impairment in the swallowing (pharyngeal) phase because the tongue plays a vital role in the process of moving foods and liquids to the back of the mouth for swallowing.

IMPAIRED CHEWING

Damage, such as weakness or partial paralysis that occurs after a stroke, may affect the ability to chew solids. Foods may collect between the cheek and the gum area (pocketing) on the affected (weak) side. A person who has suffered a stroke may bite her cheek without realizing it due to loss of sensation on the side of the body affected by the stroke.

Weakness in the lip and cheek muscles may result in foods or liquids leaking out of the weak side of her mouth or create residue on her lips. She may not realize she has foods on her mouth or that she has foods pocketed in her cheek because she doesn't feel it. She may drool during meals or between meals for similar reasons. Oral dryness may also be a problem if she takes multiple medications or is on oxygen. Lack of sufficient moisture may reduce her ability to break down foods in her mouth sufficiently for swallowing. Weakness in the soft palate (velum) may lead to liquids exiting the nose. Patients with Parkinson's disease, ALS or Multiple Sclerosis may experience liquids exiting from the nose. This is primarily caused by weakness in the soft palate (velum) and supporting muscles that help to make a tight seal when she is swallowing. Jaw impairments such as reduced jaw opening, lack of jaw control or decreased range of motion may result in a "munching" chewing pattern characterized by a tendency to chew primarily on the front teeth. This may affect how well foods are broken down and collected to form the bolus. Those afflicted with Alzheimer's disease often exhibit a "munching" chewing pattern versus a rotary chewing pattern.

PHARYNGEAL PHASE (SWALLOWING PHASE)

The structures involved in swallowing are: The throat muscles, epiglottis, true and false vocal folds (also referred to as vocal "cords") and the larynx (sometimes referred to as "voice box") valleculae and pyriform sinuses (spaces within the throat), and the hyoid bone (the tongue is anchored here). Timing is a key factor as well. It takes only a matter of seconds for a soft ball of food to reach the esophagus (tube to the stomach) once it is swallowed. Food consistency, bite size, muscle tone, muscle function, nerve function, cognitive abilities and age are factors in being able to safely swallow foods and liquids.

NORMAL

Once the swallow response is initiated, the bolus is moved to the back of the tongue in preparation for swallowing. At this point, several things happen in quick succession. A complex series of muscle contractions cause the soft palate to elevate. This seals and protects the nasal cavity and increases oral pressure to help move the foods along. The hyoid bone elevates during the swallow, raising the lower part of the tongue (attached to the hyoid bone). The base of the tongue then connects with the back of the throat (pharynx). The larynx (voice box) rises causing the epiglottis (a leaf-like cartilage structure) to flip over to protect the trachea (windpipe). All these "valves" serve to prevent foods or liquids from slipping, dripping or falling into the airway.

IMPAIRED

Primary causes of impairment in this phase are 1) poor swallow timing 2) poor coordination 3) muscle weakness or paralysis 4) poor awareness or attention. In the presence of stroke, you or the person in your care may have slower responses to swallowing. If any one of these steps is impaired for any reason, the result may be choking and or chronic aspiration pneumonia.

CHAPTER 2

Different diseases and disorders can cause a variety of chewing and swallowing problems in the elderly. General information on chewing impairments is also included under the anatomy and function section of Chapter 1. At the end of each chapter, I have included a list of diagnoses under the heading "At risk for" to help you identify problems that may point to an untreated chewing and swallowing disorder.

Symptoms of chewing or swallowing impairment may include*:
- Excessive time needed to eat
- Prolonged chewing time
- Inefficient chewing
- Coughing when eating solid foods
- Coughing when drinking
- Increased coughing with straw drinking
- Difficulty swallowing pills
- Complaints of foods "sticking in his throat"
- Feeling like he has a "lump" in his throat, also called "globus sensation"
- Runny nose
- Red eyes
- Avoiding foods
- Fear of choking
- Often clearing his throat while eating
- Wet sounding voice, particularly if speaking when eating
- Coughing at meals
- Choking episodes
- Intermittent temperature spikes, usually after meals and then subsides
- Lethargy
- Vomiting
- Gagging
- Producing large amounts of phlegm or mucus
- Weight loss

*(If these are new symptoms or have gotten worse, notify the physician immediately).

A WORD ON COUGHING

Coughing is <u>always</u> a reflex to prevent choking or to rid the lungs of an irritant. The irritant may be of non-food origin such as post-nasal drip or saliva, however, if it occurs regularly at meals and after the meal, <u>be suspicious</u>. It may indicate that foods or liquids are entering the lungs. This can lead to aspiration pneumonia over time. Chronic coughing at night may be a sign of unmanaged reflux. Contacting the physician is recommended if any of these symptoms occur.

IMPAIRMENTS BY DISEASE BY OR DISORDER

This section addresses key diseases that affect the nerves and muscles involved in chewing and swallowing.

STROKE
ORAL PHASE (Chewing):

- Often exhibits signs of oral dysarthria (weak tongue, lip, cheek muscles), typically on the side of the body affected by the stroke.

- Typically one side of the face will be weaker than the other.

- The body is wired to prevent complete unilateral (one-sided) damage, therefore, a stroke in the left hemisphere of the brain will result in weakness or paralysis on the right side of the body and vice versa.

- Weakness in the tongue, lips and cheeks (a condition called dysarthria) may cause pocketing of foods (i.e. foods tucked in the channels between the cheeks and gums/teeth).
- It is possible for her to have weakness on both sides if she has had multiple strokes.

- Weakness in the tongue may make result foods falling from the mouth, residue on the lips, foods scattered along the tongue due to poor ability to form the bolus (soft ball of chewed foods).
- She may bite her cheek while chewing and she may or may not realize it depending on the degree of sensation she has in the affected (impaired or weak) area.
- She may drool during meals and between meals.
- Dentures may not fit as they did prior to the stroke. This may be a long-standing issue that is now made worse because the muscles and nerves are weak or it may be due to weight loss related to illness. The absence of natural teeth or dentures may dramatically affect the individual's ability to break down foods for safe chewing, swallowing and effective digestion.
- Her mouth may be excessively dry due to medications, which may reduce her ability to moisten and break down foods properly. Ask your doctor about over-the-counter Biotene or other products to improve moisture in the mouth.
- She may ignore foods or liquids placed on her affected side, even failing to eat foods on that side of her plate. She may not even realize this food is there if she has visual field impairment from her stroke (example: if the right side is paralyzed, she may not turn to look at the right side due to lack of normal vision on that side).
- Changing food texture may be required. More on diet modification will be discussed in Chapter 3.

PHARYNGEAL PHASE (SWALLOWING)

- May exhibit dysarthria (muscle weakness) of the throat muscles.
- One side of the throat may be weaker than the other. A person with problems swallowing may not sense foods or liquids traveling down the weak or paralyzed side and fail to swallow quickly enough to prevent penetration (foods or liquids entering the airway and dropping to the level of the vocal cords) or aspiration (foods or liquids passing through the vocal cords into the windpipe).
- The muscles that lift the larynx (voice box) may be weak reducing full range of motion of the larynx.
- Lack of full range of motion of the larynx during swallowing may result in incomplete excursion (forward movement) of the larynx.
- Inadequate excursion of the larynx may lead to inadequate closure of the vocal cords over the airway.
- The epiglottis (leaf-like cartilage structure that helps protect the windpipe) may not fully invert to shield the airway.
- Unilateral (one side) weakness in a vocal cord may prevent the vocal cords from closing completely allowing foods or liquids to drip or fall into the airway.
- Foods or liquids may pool in the spaces in the throat and drip into the airway even after the meal is over.
- May experience chronic diagnosis of bronchitis, asthma, pneumonia

At Risk For:

- Choking
- Weight Loss
- Oral lacerations caused by biting his tongue or the inside of his cheeks due to decreased sensation. If he doesn't sense or remove food residue on his

lips, this may be an indicator that he won't feel it if he bites his tongue or cheek.

- Urinary Tract Infections if he doesn't drink a sufficient amount of fluids daily.
- Aspiration Pneumonia
- Chronic Congestion
- Dental issues if he has natural teeth and his mouth is excessively dry due to medications or if he neglects oral care on this side due to lack of awareness and sensation.

PARKINSON'S DISEASE

Those who suffer with Parkinson's disease will exhibit slow movements in general, due to weakness and rigidity. The parent or spouse may have difficulty initiating (starting) a task. The oral phase of swallowing is typically affected by slow oral movements, difficulty getting the "chewing" started, reduced range of chewing, reduced tongue strength, slow swallow response and weak throat muscles, all which may cause:

Oral Phase:
- Signs of oral dysarthria (weak tongue, lip, cheek muscles
- Decreased rotary chew (normal chewing motion); tends to "munch" foods
- Decreased ability to form a cohesive bolus (chewed ball of food that sticks together)
- Decreased ability to move the bolus to the back of the throat for swallowing
- Pocketing (foods tucked inside the cheek and gums)
- Drooling and difficulty
- Inability to chew some solid food such as meats and harder vegetables
- Inability to control thin liquids
- Weak, soft voice, sometimes barely audible

Pharyngeal Phase:
- Delayed swallow

- Wet Voice
- Temperature spikes after meals
- Weak cough, or coughing seen at or after meals
- Throat clearing
- Chronic congestion
- Chronic diagnosis of bronchitis, asthma, pneumonia

At Risk For:
- Choking
- Weight Loss
- Urinary Tract Infections if she doesn't drink a sufficient amount of fluids daily
- Aspiration Pneumonia
- Chronic Congestion

ALZHEIMER'S DISEASE AND OTHER COGNITIVE IMPAIRMENTS

Alzheimer's Disease, senile dementia or other types of brain damage such as a head injury or surgeries involving the brain often come with an overall decline in cognitive function. Cognitive loss may lead to difficulty eating and drinking safely over time. An individual may lose his ability to sequence steps, focus and sustain his attention or show poor judgment and decreased safety awareness. Here are some symptoms to look for if a chewing or swallowing problem is suspected:

Oral Phase:
- Excessive chewing for several minutes without swallowing, or failure to swallow without being instructed to do so.
- Pockets foods on one side of the mouth without swallowing.
- Packs his mouth with several bites and continuing to chew without swallowing.
- Removes partially chewed foods from his mouth that are hard to chewing.

- Spits particles of food into the air or on the floor (likely because he doesn't recognize the texture as food).
- Attempting to eat non-food items such as cloth napkins, paper or plastic products, or other non-food items.**
- Engage in talking or calling out when eating which increases choking risk

** He may also experience problems with self-feeding and use utensils incorrectly or engage in odd behavior such as pouring juice on his toast due to confusion or difficulty remembering the correct steps involved.

Pharyngeal Phase:
- Delayed Swallow
- Coughing or choking at meals
- Temperature spikes
- Weight loss
- Food avoidance (because the foods are too difficult to eat, he may not recognize foods, or he may have lost his sense of taste)
- Wet voice
- Throat clearing
- Chronic congestion
- Chronic diagnosis of bronchitis, asthma, pneumonia

At Risk For:
- Weight loss
- Choking
- Pneumonia
- Failure to thrive if refusing foods and liquids

ALS (Amyotrophic lateral sclerosis or Lou Gehrig's Disease)
ALS is characterized by muscle tissue atrophy (wasting or withering of the muscles). While ALS speech and swallowing symptoms appear to be similar to multiple sclerosis, they stem from different sources. In ALS, the nerve cells die in the brain and spine die often resulting in a shorter life span. The

17

individual may eventually lose her ability to speak and is often unable to breathe on her own because the brain cannot communicate with or engage the muscles of the body. Speech is often slow, nasal sounding and slurred.

Oral Phase:
- Oral weakness
- Slow mastication
- Decreased range of motion when chewing
- Pocketing
- Difficulty forming a cohesive bolus (soft ball of food)
- Difficulty moving foods to the back of the mouth to swallow (oral transit)
- Drooling or poor saliva control
- Speech may be slurred, slow or halting which is a clue about how the tongue and mouth muscles are working

Pharyngeal Phase:
- Delayed swallow
- Reduced strength of swallow
- Reduced coordination of swallow
- Globus sensation (feeling like foods are "sticking" in the throat) or feeling as if there is a "lump" in the throat
- Coughing while eating or drinking or immediately after eating or drinking
- Choking episode(s)
- Increased fatigue when eating
- Inability to eat by mouth due to problems with vocal fold (cord) function*

*Neurological problems that affect the nerves used in speech and breath support will most likely affect the swallowing abilities as well. If the vocal cords do not open and close sufficiently for breathing and speaking, they may not close enough to prevent foods and liquids from entering the windpipe, and eventually, the lungs.

At Risk For:
- Chronic upper respiratory infections
- Aspiration pneumonia
- Choking
- Dehydration and malnutrition due to chewing and swallowing impairments
- Weight loss
- Failure to thrive

MULTIPLE SCLEROSIS

Multiple Sclerosis (MS) is characterized by the inability of nerves to communicate (synapse) with one another due to loss of myelin (protective tissue) around the nerves. Speech may be affected, but unlike individuals with ALS, the patient diagnosed with MS typically has a longer life span and may not develop severe symptoms for many years.

Oral Phase:
- Oral weakness
- Slow mastication
- Decreased range of motion when chewing
- Pocketing
- May have difficulty with saliva control
- Difficulty forming a cohesive bolus (ball of chewed food)
- Difficulty moving foods to the back of the mouth for swallowing (impaired oral transit)
- Speech may be slurred, slow, or halting which is a clue about how the tongue and mouth muscles are working

Pharyngeal Phase:
- Coughing while eating drinking or immediately after
- Choking episode(s)
- Globus sensation (feeling as if food is "stuck" or there is a lump in his throat)
- Increased fatigue when eating

At Risk For:
- Choking
- Weight loss
- Chronic lung infections
- Aspiration pneumonia
- UTI if he doesn't drink enough liquids

CHAPTER 3

DIET MODIFICATION

What is diet modification? In a nutshell, it is changing the texture and consistency of foods by mechanically grinding, mashing, blending or cooking them in a way that makes them easier to chew and swallow. Modified diets do not include raw foods or foods that are hard to chew or pose choking hazards such as steak, hotdogs, nuts, popcorn, or hard candy.

MECHANICALLY ALTERED FOODS, THIN AND THICKENED LIQUIDS

Simply put, a person with dysphagia may need to change her food consistency to make it easier to chew and safer to swallow. When I recommend this as a practitioner, I encounter considerable resistance to the idea of chopping or grinding up meats and vegetables or adding commercial thickener to drinks. It's not surprising. At this point, an individual with swallowing problems may have lost a considerable degree of independence in other functional areas as well. Perhaps she cannot walk without assistance or even toilet or bathe herself any longer. She may have lost her ability to drive and is now dependent on others. It often feels like insult to injury for her, and those who care for her, when she can no longer safely eat foods that she enjoys.

Factor in cultural and social considerations associated with no longer being able to eat the way other people do, and it is understandable that an individual who now has to eat pureed foods or drink thickened liquids may develop depression or refuse to eat and drink altogether which can put her in a downward spiral medically.

Though modified foods are not always appealing to consider, refusing to eat or drink modified foods and liquids or choosing to eat foods or drink liquids that are not safe may lead to pneumonia, urinary tract infections, malnutrition, dehydration or result in choking and early death.

HOW YOU TALK MATTERS!

Over the 17 years of my practice, I have heard well meaning, loving family members and dedicated nurse's aides describe someone in their care as being "like a baby again." Though the level of swallowing impairment and dementia may produce behaviors that seem child-like, the adult swallowing structures are much different than that of an infant. Reclining an infant slightly for feeding may be appropriate, however this is never the case with an adult. An individual who is bedridden—whether he lives in his home or a nursing home—may be at higher risk for aspiration related respiratory illness and choking due if he is not elevated to a proper sitting position during meals. In fact, positioning is so critical for safety that the number one cause of aspiration is poor positioning followed by lack of sufficient oral care, incorrect safe diet consistency and being fed large bites or sips of liquids too quickly. Positioning will be further discussed in Chapter 4.

I have also heard any number of inappropriate words used to describe a pureed meal WHILE THE INDIVIDUAL WAS EATING IT. Imagine that the only foods you can eat are pureed foods. Your husband/wife/daughter or nurse's aide comes into the room and proceeds to talk about how unappealing, disgusting or sickening the food looks. Would you want to eat it? As an SLP working in nursing homes, I have heard any number of staff and family members discouraged the poor resident who has to eat pureed foods for safety put that very food down or even compare it to "dog poop" or "pig slop." Talking this way about foods an impaired person has to eat may serve the ego of the person doing it, but it does nothing to promote eating or safety for the individual faced with 1) eating pureed foods or 2) risking choking and pneumonia if he doesn't eat pureed foods. In this scenario, the individual usually does not eat well and loses weight which compromises his overall health or he refuses the safe consistency and elects to eat solids sometimes resulting in chronic pneumonia or choking episodes. In some cases, the wrong consistency, while having more appeal, may also result in weight loss because the patient avoids foods due to fear of choking.

Resistance to modified moods is typically made by family members who feel guilt, frustration or sadness that their loved is losing a skill they see as both simple and basic: the act of eating. It hits us at our emotional core to realize that our parent or spouse may no longer be able to eat his favorite foods or drink his coffee without thickening powder. Paid caregivers may argue or resist a modified consistency for those in their care because they feel affection for their patient, worry that she is not eating the altered foods or because she is vocal about her dislike of modified foods.

It's important to remember whom these changes affect. This is about the person in your care and what he or she needs to do to be safe. Positive language and a supportive, encouraging attitude changes everything. You have the power to create an atmosphere of acceptance or rejection. I guarantee that negative comments will not yield positive results with regard to safer swallowing and adequate eating.

CAN I USE BABY FOOD?

The chore of pureeing foods is not always easy for working caregivers. For more alert individuals with dysphagia who still have the ability to manage some tasks and want to prepare their own meals or snacks, pureeing a meal may not be an option for them. In these cases, it is perfectly fine to use baby foods to bridge the meal gap for an adult who no longer has the ability to chew or has significant chewing or swallowing problems, but we need to remember that he is not an infant.

If he is aware of what is happening, it is likely that he will feel embarrassed about eating puree foods if the people around him describe his food as "baby food" particularly if this is discussed in an insensitive manner. Even though a dysphagia sufferer may now be very confused, hard of hearing or perhaps, nonverbal, it is neither dignified, nor respectful, to compare an adult to an infant. Speaking negatively about his food may result in poor eating or prompt him to choose unmodified foods that increase his choking or pneumonia risk.

If you choose to use baby food, check with the physician and a dietitian to ensure your loved one or your patient is getting balanced and appropriate nutrition. Please put the food in a regular dish the same as you would for anyone you would serve a meal. Feeding an adult from a baby food jar is a dignity issue. If it would embarrass you, don't do it to them!

We must put ourselves in the individual's shoes and preserve his or her dignity as much as possible by being sensitive about how we handle these changes.

Below are some suggestions about how to encourage those with swallowing problems to accept modified foods:

- Use positive language to describe foods, such as "This smells great!" or "Look, Dad, we have _____ for lunch today."

- Season foods to increase flavor and appeal. Keep dietary restrictions such as "no salt" in mind when seasoning foods.

- Eat with your parent or spouse. Eating is a social activity. Nursing home patients left in their rooms or in bed often have the worst track record for eating well.

- Isolation decreases the amount of foods an individual will eat. Even if he prefers to eat in front of the television, he will likely eat more if someone sits with him and eats as well.

- If he is eating pureed foods, eat foods that are similar in consistency if possible such as applesauce, pudding or soup. If your food resembles his food, he may be more inclined to eat a modified diet. That's not to say you can't eat foods that are appropriate for you, but if you are visiting someone with chewing or swallowing difficulties, eating something similar to his diet consistency during the visit may improve his acceptance of his diet.

Food quality and preparation will vary among institutions. It is not possible for a facility to season large-scale meals for each individual taste. If your relative or patient is in a long-term care facility, bringing in the occasional home cooked pureed food may go a long way in increasing his acceptance of modified foods. Bringing in foods does not have to be elaborate or expensive. Even simple foods such as homemade mashed potatoes have a different taste than those made commercially and, when added to the meal tray, may improve the patient's desire to eat.

If you live with someone who has a chewing or swallowing impairment, you can modify foods from your own meals to a consistency that he can safely eat (see pureed foods below for more ideas on making purees palatable).

MODIFIED FOODS

PUREED FOODS

Pureed foods require no chewing and are blended until they are smooth and free of any lumps or solid texture. Mashed potatoes, yogurt (without fruit), applesauce, and pudding are a few examples of natural purees. Home cooked purees are quite simple to make using a baby food cooker, regular blender or an individual blender such as the ones that are used to make smoothies. Prices and descriptions detailed below are those listed at the time this book was written and subject to change.

Though I am not endorsing any particular product, I have listed a few ideas to give readers a place to start, particularly for those who are completely in the dark about preparing pureed foods.

I have personally used variations on the Magic Bullet and the Nutri-Bullet with good success, though these machines do not completely "puree" raw foods, they will thoroughly puree banana, berries, raw apples or raw spinach, but may not break down kale or other fiberous raw vegetables sufficiently for someone on a puree diet. Fiberous vegetables will puree more easily if you cook them before you puree them. The Nutri-Bullet comes with a second "grinding" attachment that allows you to mill (pulverize) seeds and nuts into a powdery form.

Williams and Sonoma offers The Beaba BabyCook Baby Food Maker, a French baby-food cooker. The product description on the label states that this cooker "steams, warms, defrosts and blends foods to a puree in about 15 minutes while "retaining all the vitamins and minerals" in the foods. Beaba also makes companion freezer trays and storage containers for food preparation ahead of time. At approximately $115, it is slightly more expensive than other options such as a regular blender.

A food processor, such as a Cuisinart, may be more versatile, cost effective and sufficiently puree foods from the family meal.

A word on flavor: As we age, our taste buds may not be as sensitive to varied flavors. Bland foods may decrease the likelihood that the patient will eat well unless this has always been his preference. If you are pureeing foods at home, consider these options (if the physician and/or dietitian approves based on individual tolerance of salt and other seasonings):

- Use broth or milk instead of water to thin sticky or thick purees, such as pureed macaroni and cheese.
- Cook foods in the normal method (e.g. baked chicken, cooked meat sauce for spaghetti) and blend it with small amounts of broth (or water if the dish already has salt in it) to thin it. Avoid sticky foods. Be careful not to add too much liquid as this may make the dish too thin
- Consider no-salt options to liven up foods such as herbs: rosemary, oregano, thyme, garlic powder, onion powder, Papa and Mama dash, lemon, dill, sage, and many other seasonings. Consult with a dietitian for more ideas and recommendations, particularly if there are cultural considerations regarding herbs and spices such as cumin, curry, pepper and spicier options.
- If the person in your care can safely drink thin liquids, milk or juice may be used to "slurry" or soften cakes, muffins and cookies into a puree. These items should not have any nuts, seeds, or raisins in them. Example: Put a soft piece of cake in a dish, add milk to the bottom and let it soak into the cake. Use a spoon or fork to agitate or mash the cake and milk together. This can be done successfully with donuts, too, as long as you allow the donut to soak up the milk and soften so that it

can be "stirred" into a puree. The liquid and cake or donut can also be pureed in a blender.

- Using similar flavored liquids increases palatability. For example, apple muffins or cakes can be softened with apple juice to help retain the apple flavor.
- If the individual is consuming thickened liquids, you can soften desserts in the same manner, just use thickened liquids and prepare in the same manner described above for thin liquids.

COMMERCIALLY PREPARED BABY FOOD

If you are unable to prepare foods due to time, budget or other constraints, baby foods are a good option because they are nutritious, affordable and convenient. You can also add seasonings to baby foods to increase their palatability. Check with a physician or dietitian to ensure that the vitamin and mineral content of these foods are appropriate for your parent, spouse or patient. If you choose to feed baby or infant foods, please remove them from the baby food jars and serve them in the same dishes you would use to serve any member of the family. It is simply not respectful or dignified to feed an adult from a baby food jar.

MECHANICAL SOFT FOODS

This diet is not to be confused with a soft diet recommended by a physician, often due to gastric surgery or gastric issues.

Mechanical soft foods are foods that are easy to chew. This diet consistency works well for individuals with missing teeth and those who are edentulous (have no teeth and do not wear dentures) if they do not have trouble swallowing.

Mechanical soft foods have been soft cooked and cut or diced into pieces no larger than one half inch. Meats are ground, shredded or diced into small cubes or soft, thin pieces. This consistency does not allow any raw, hard, chewy, tough or whole foods (see REGULAR consistency). Mechanical soft foods should have skins or rinds removed before or after cooking as they may pose a chewing or choking problem for a person with difficulty swallowing.

EXAMPLES OF MECHANICAL SOFT FOODS:
- Macaroni and Cheese or other soft cooked noodles
- Soft cooked chicken (steamed or baked)
- Soft cooked fish without bones
- Soft breads, cakes or pastries
- Soft cookies without nuts or raisins
- The inside of a baked potato
- Egg salad sandwich filling (without onions or celery, whites diced small)
- Soft fruits such as diced canned peaches and pears.

Meats and vegetables often pose a greater chewing and choking problem than other foods. Meats are primarily muscle and stringy connective tissue while vegetables are high in fiber. String beans, zucchini, succotash or combinations of corn, lima beans and other side dishes with skins and rinds may require considerable effort to chew, even after cooking.

Prolonged chewing may increase his fatigue with eating. If he gets tired because eating is now "work" he may give up and eat less. If the vegetable side dishes are a problem, serving a combination of consistencies may help. For example, a meal may consist of a mechanical soft entrée like soft cooked fish or an egg salad sandwich with pureed sides such as squash or mashed potatoes or vegetables that have been cooked and then pureed.

If you need more information on what is or isn't a mechanical soft food, ask your health care professional for a list of foods that may be allowed or go online and search "mechanical soft foods." Remember that your physician, speech pathologist and dietitian are excellent resources for providing information on what is a safe and balanced diet for each consistency.

CHOPPED FOODS

This consistency varies, but typically, foods are cut into small bite-sized pieces. All foods may be chopped or chopping may be limited only to problem foods.

REGULAR FOODS

Any food that requires considerable chewing or has a hard, tough (such as beef jerky), or chewy consistency is a regular diet consistency food. Foods in this category are not modified but served as cooked or packaged.

EXAMPLES

Steak, fried chicken, potato chips, nuts, raisins, popcorn, bagels, English muffins, submarine sandwiches with layers of meats and other toppings, taco shells, jerky, soups with chunks of meat, most raw vegetables and fruits (e.g. pineapple chunks or rings, orange slices, apples) with the exception of bananas.

LIQUIDS

Liquids present a special problem for people with a swallowing disorder because they travel very fast making them more difficult to control. Adding a natural food to increase bulk or a commercial thickener to a liquid can slow down the rate in which it travels making it easier and safer to swallow.

Commercial thickening agents come in gel or powdered form and work in a similar way. You can use any thickening agent that works for your budget and is easy to find.

To better understand how to thicken liquids, you can view a Resource ThickenUp demonstration at http://www.youtube.com/watch?v=e4RA2CJ6czU. It is imperative that you, the caregiver, learn how to appropriately thicken liquids and be able to distinguish between thin, nectar or honey-thickened liquid in order to offer the correct, safe liquid consistency to those in your care. Consuming liquids that are too thin can cause pneumonia. (See Chapter 4 for more on Aspiration Pneumonia).

The flip side of this coin is that, while over-thickening a drink because you're concerned about the safety of your spouse or parent may seem like the best idea to prevent pneumonia, it can lead to dehydration if he isn't drinking enough fluids. If he needs nectar-thickened liquids and you're providing him with honey-thickened liquids unnecessarily, he may not drink enough. An individual receiving thickened liquids may need to drink extra fluids to ensure he remains hydrated. If he is on a fluid restriction, consult his physician for advice as to how to best meet his individual needs.

In some cases, those who need thickened liquids can still manage a little cold water even if they aspirate it (see "free water" section at the end of this chapter). Care must be taken when providing "free" or thin water for those on thickened liquid restrictions.

THIN LIQUIDS
Obvious thin liquids are water, milk, soda pop and other carbonated beverages, alcoholic beverages such as beer, wine and liquor, supplements such as Boost or other nutritional drinks, coffee, orange juice, apple and cranberry juices. Less obvious thin liquids are: broth, soup bases, ice cream, milkshakes, and Jell-O.

Many of my patients and their families are puzzled by the fact that ice cream is frozen, so "how can it be a thin liquid?" Body temperature and saliva break down ice cream, milk shakes and Jell-O. By the time the mouth has warmed the foods and mixed them with saliva, they behave similarly to water or other thin liquids. If a liquid flows quickly, it is a thin liquid.

A word on straws: If your patient is drinking through a straw and coughing (a sign that the liquids are entering his lungs) the straw may be the culprit. Straws allow for larger amounts of liquids to be taken into the mouth at one time, often decreasing swallowing control. It is possible he may be able to take small sips of thin liquid from a cup and swallow it safely. More on safety strategies in Chapter 5.

NECTAR-THICKENED LIQUIDS

Nectar thickened fluids are those that have been thickened to the consistency of nectar syrup such as that in fruit cocktail.

Most pharmacies will have one or two brands that usually have the word "thick" in the title. All brands work in a similar fashion. The primary difference in brands is price, palatability and the amount of time it takes for them to thicken the liquid. You should use the brand that works best for your budget. Examples of thickening agents are ThickenUp or Thick-It.

Tolerance of powdered thickeners is sometimes a problem if the thickener is not sufficiently mixed with the liquid. Using a regular blender for large quantities of fluid or a hand-held blender for single servings will create a smoother, more palatable drink. Hand-held blending wands sell from around $11 to $50. If you are mixing several glasses or a pitcher of liquid and refrigerating them, you may want to use a regular blender.

Using a blender may help to reduce grains in the drink and make it smooth, however all thickeners can be mixed using a regular spoon. Directions are provided on the label of the can for a specific size glass (4 ounces or 8 ounces). Your physician, speech pathologist or dietitian can advise you what type of thickener to purchase. A speech pathologist or dietitian can teach you how to prepare nectar-thickened liquids.

Premixed thickened liquids are available for purchase from food supply companies. While these products are more palatable, they are also more expensive. For example: Six (8) ounce boxes of Resource lemon-flavored honey-thickened water sell for $9.99. Resource brand is a Nestle foods company. Amazon.com lists 4-ounce containers of honey-thick Thick and Easy water (24 per package) for $15.38 (as of the writing of this book—prices may change) with no shipping charges if the purchaser has an account that qualifies for no shipping.

Another option is using natural foods when possible to thicken items particularly to improve acceptance of a thicker beverage. Example: Yogurt can be mixed with milk products to increase their thickness naturally. Soups can be thickened with potato flakes or instant rice flakes (baby rice is a good option) as long as the product does not cause chunks, lumps or particles that make chewing necessary for those on puree foods.

HONEY-THICKENED LIQUIDS
Honey-thickened liquids do not contain honey. Honey-thickened is merely a descriptive term to give you an idea about how thick the liquid should be. Honey-thickened liquids flow more slowly from the cup than nectar. To get an idea of what a particular thickened liquid should look like, I use the "spoon test" to educate family members and nurse's aides. This isn't a hard and fast rule, but it gives a visual idea about what a thickened liquid looks like. Place a plastic spoon in a cup of thickened liquid. If it stands upright briefly before it falls to the side, it's honey-thickened. If the spoon falls over immediately, it's likely nectar thick consistency. If it remains standing, it is likely pudding thick.

I have observed both CNA's (certified nursing assistants) and family members put less than the recommended scoop into a drink and let it settle to the bottom because they thought the end result was "too thick." This will result in the drink remaining a thin consistency. Making the drink thicker (and safer) is the reason for adding the thickening agent. Adding insufficient thickener to the drink or letting it settle to the bottom is a waste of money and does nothing to promote safety.

PUDDING THICKENED LIQUIDS
Just as the name implies, this liquid is as thick as pudding. It should be consumed with a spoon, as it is not possible to

actually "drink" pudding-thickened liquids. I seldom recommend this level of thickness unless the patient in my care has a profound swallowing disorder and is not able to manage anything else. If your spouse or parent has been advised to consume pudding thickened liquids due to a severe or profound swallowing problem or recurrent pneumonias, he may need to consume extra servings per day to prevent dehydration. Ask the appropriate healthcare professionals caring for advice about this and clear it with his physician.

FREE WATER
Even though they may aspirate it, some individuals are given "free" or thin cold water under very specific conditions to prevent dehydration (see Chapter 4 for more on Aspiration).

There are STRICT applications for the administration of cold water in dysphagia patients and you must consult with your doctor, and, if you are working with one, the speech pathologist, prior to initiating this practice.

CONDITIONS FOR ALLOWING FREE COLD WATER are listed below. Water is natural to the body and does not cause chemical injury in the lungs if provided appropriately and in small amounts. **Other thin beverages may cause chemical injury to the lungs and result in the development of pneumonia if aspirated**.

Administration of free water
- The patient's mouth should be clean, with teeth or dentures brushed prior to drinking cold thin water.
- No foods, medications are consumed with the cold thin water, and no other liquids are allowed.
- Remember, some of this water "may" enter the lungs so you don't want drops of juice or coffee, or particles of foods or pills carried along with it.
- She should be sitting upright in a chair
- She should NOT use a straw

- She should sit up for about 30 minutes after eating or drinking any foods or liquids, including cold, thin water.
- If she exhibits excessive coughing, produces mucus or becomes congested with thin water, please call the physician and report this and ask for advice about whether or not to continue.

ABUSE OF FREE WATER
Large amounts of cold water consumed while reclined, or with foods or medications or using a straw may result in development of pneumonia. Substitution of any liquids other than cold water as described above may also result in pneumonia.

CHAPTER 4

ASPIRATION

Aspiration pneumonia occurs when foods or liquids enter the lungs. Below is a series of precautions and strategies to ensure the safety of a spouse, parent or patient at risk for aspiration pneumonia due to chewing or swallowing problems.

ASPIRATION PRECAUTIONS

WAYS TO PREVENT CHOKING AND PNEUMONIA

Many strategies we use to prevent choking and aspiration are common sense, however when an individual is paralyzed or has dementia which increases the physical and emotional energy required to care for them, it is tempting to eliminate steps in order to save work or time. This is common in institutional setting such as skilled nursing facilities where the workload is often heavy with insufficient staff to perform that work. If your loved one is in a skilled nursing facility, you may need to advocate firmly about using these strategies to ensure his safety with meals, snacks and medication passes. If he is at home, these strategies will help to ensure he is as safe as possible when eating or drinking.

STRATEGIES
- Prepare the correct food and liquid consistencies.
- If he is on a strict puree and thickened liquid diet, do not give him foods with "texture" such as bits of fruit in yogurt or diced or mashed foods with lumps.
- Do not offer him thin liquids even to swallow medications. Medications can be swallowed with thickened fluids or added, one at a time, to yogurt, applesauce or pudding for safer swallowing. Please

check with your pharmacist before you break or crush a medication. Some medications are formulated for slow release in the body.

- Brush his teeth or dentures and clean his mouth before breakfast and after subsequent meals. Soak dentures in a denture cleaning solution each night to ensure cleanliness. A clean mouth is essential to avoiding aspiration. Even if your patient or loved one doesn't have teeth, he still has bacteria in his mouth when he wakes up in the morning.
- Use a denture adhesive to prevent dentures from rolling around in his mouth or falling down when he chews. Fighting his dentures while trying to chew his food may increase his choking risk, but it will certainly reduce his ability to adequately chew his food.
- Seat him in a regular chair or his wheelchair at a table for all meals.

CORRECT POSITION
The individual's back and trunk should be upright, with bottom scooted as far back in the seat as possible. His feet should be on the floor or foot rests if he sits in a wheelchair.

INCORRECT POSITION
No one should eat in a reclined position, least of all those with swallowing problems. If his bottom is scooted forward, he may slide out of the chair. His head and shoulders should not rest on a pillow or the back of the chair.

FOR BEDBOUND PATIENTS
- It is unsafe to eat lying down or reclined.
- If he doesn't have the trunk muscles to sit erect in the chair, you can use pillows to improve his posture.
- Remember, mealtime is not the place to "get comfortable" as he would for a nap. He needs to be as alert as possible, sitting up and participating in his meal if he is able.

- Supervise meals to ensure he uses strategies such as tucking his chin when he swallows or taking small sips and bites.
- Have him sit up for a minimum of half an hour after meals to improve digestion and reduce risk of reflux aspiration.

BREATHING PROBLEMS

Because we have to hold our breath to swallow, this can create fatigue in an individual who already struggles to breathe. Individuals with breathing problems tend to eat large amounts of food rapidly before they tire which increases his choking and aspiration risk. Some patients will stop eating after a few bites due to fatigue which may impact nutrition. An individual with COPD (Chronic Obstructive Pulmonary Disease) may better tolerate several small meals per day than three larger ones.

PARALYSIS OR WEAKNESS

If your parent or spouse has paralysis or weakness on one side of his face, place foods for chewing on the opposite side to reduce the risk of biting the inside of his cheek or tongue on the weak side. If he has seen a speech pathologist, and an exercise program has been established, encourage him to follow the plan. This plan may improve his strength and overall tolerance of foods and liquids as well as reduce his choking aspiration risk.

CHAPTER 5

TESTS AND TREATMENT FOR DYSPHAGIA

There are three (3) primary methods of evaluating swallow function:

(1) A bedside or tableside swallowing evaluation
(2) A radiology procedure that involves the individual drinking barium
(3) An endoscope placed through the nose to determine swallow function and tolerance of foods and liquids during a meal or snack

Let's take a look at the different types of swallowing evaluations (tests).

SUBJECTIVE SWALLOWING EVALUATION

A subjective evaluation is one that relies on the speech pathologists expertise but does not involve x-rays or the insertion of scopes. During a bedside or tableside swallowing evaluation, the speech pathologist observes the patient eat and drink using foods and liquids from his meal or snack. If he is in a hospital or skilled nursing facility, this evaluation is typically performed at the bedside or in an appropriate dining area. For those patients still living at home, a home health based speech language pathologist (SLP) can also assess the patient with a snack or meal using available foods from your kitchen. Once the evaluation is completed, the SLP then makes the appropriate recommendations regarding what consistencies are safe as well as strategies to improve safety and reduce choking and aspiration risks. The bedside swallowing evaluation is highly accurate due to the education and experience of the SLP, however, there are times when it is difficult to pinpoint the problem if there are a host of other health issues that mask or confuse the symptoms. A subjective test may yield inconclusive results if he is medically fragile or has a higher than usual risk for choking and aspiration. Individuals with a history of chronic pneumonia, an inability to tolerate any food or liquid consistencies during a bedside swallowing evaluation, or a parent who has been eating through a feeding tube for some time should have objective testing due to their level of risk. To that end, the SLP may not believe it is safe to offer foods and liquids or may recommend further testing to define his condition or confirm the results of the bedside swallow evaluation.

OBJECTIVE SWALLOWING EVALUATION

An objective test is one that uses instruments to allow the speech pathologist to visually determine what happens when the patient eats and drinks. It is possible to pass an objective test and later have problems at home, but this is not a common occurrence. Problems typically develop when the individual does not follow the recommendations. Let's take a look at the two most commonly used tests.

Videofluoroscopic Swallow Study (VFSS) or Modified Barium Swallow Study (MBSS)

The VFSS or MBSS is typically performed through outpatient services at a local hospital radiology department. The patient sits in a chair that is designed to provide optimal positioning and viewing of his head and neck. He is presented with various consistencies of thin and thick barium as well as food items with barium paste. The barium paste is necessary so that the foods and liquids can be seen during the procedure. The speech pathologist instructs the patient to take sips or bites, or in some cases, may feed the patient. The radiologist x-rays the patient as he chews and swallows, typically for only a few seconds at a time. The radiologist turns on the machine only when the patient is actively drinking, chewing or swallowing. The speech pathologist may instruct your parent or spouse to try different techniques such as tucking his chin or coughing at certain times to improve his swallow function.

The procedure is videotaped as part of the medical record and may be referred to for further analysis and education after the study is concluded. To watch a real-time videofluoroscopy (x-ray image) please visit http://www.youtube.com/watch?v=jr2CuFRCsP8.* In this example, you can clearly see the landmarks, listen to the directions from the speech pathologist and see an example of aspiration. *As of the writing of this book, the image was still available.

FEES (Fiberoptic or Flexible Endoscopic Evaluation of Swallow)
A scope is passed through the patient's nose and hangs just above the vocal cords. The patient eats and drinks normally while the speech pathologist views the study on a monitor and records the procedure. To view an endoscopic swallow of an individual with normal swallowing please visit http://www.youtube.com/watch?v=l8elCovpb28.* As you can see during the procedure, the camera portion of the scope is "whited out" during the swallow.

OBJECTIVE STUDIES: WHICH TEST IS BETTER?
Choosing the right test for your loved one depends on the type of information you need and the severity and nature of the problem. It also depends on the individual's cognitive and physical ability to participate in the study.

There are risks and benefits with both forms of testing. For many years, the Videofluroscopic Swallow Study (VFSS, also referred to as the Modified Barium Swallow Study or MBSS) has been thought to be the gold standard for assessing swallowing difficulties because it measures the path of the foods or liquids from the moment they enter the mouth until they are swallowed, but direct view of the anatomy is not possible. Foods and liquids must be mixed with barium in order to be visible during the assessment.

*As of the writing of this book, these images were still available.

Recently, the Flexible or Fiberoptic Endoscopic Evaluation of Swallow (FEES) has gained favor with SLP's. The FEES enables the speech pathologist to directly view the anatomy of the patient, and to determine tolerance of liquids and solids in a different manner, however, the FEES cannot measure what is actually happening "during" the swallow because the act of swallowing blocks the view of the bolus. Research indicates that both tests are close in identifying various degrees of dysphagia.

A WORD ON IMAGING CENTERS

In recent years, some physicians have begun to refer patients to "imaging centers" rather than hospital radiology departments. This development is likely based on the lengthy wait to get an appointment with the speech pathologist and the radiologist for a VFSS study as well as a lack of understanding about the information needed from an objective test to identify the nature of the dysphagia and effectively manage the disorder.

The goal of a VFSS is to determine what type of foods or liquids the patient can manage and under what conditions. Without a speech pathologist available to try different food consistencies, and examine ways to get the foods and liquids to go down properly, you may leave not knowing if he is able to safely eat solid foods.

While an imaging center may be perfect if you have a sprained ankle or need a mammogram or an MRI, it is not, in my clinical experience, ideal for patients with dysphagia. Imaging staff is not specifically trained to know what to look for in patients with swallowing disorders with regard to management of solids. They use varying degrees of barium liquids or paste but (at the time of this writing) do not trial solid foods. They often use the language "pass" or "fail" as a determination about swallowing function because their focus is black and white: aspiration or no aspiration. Dysphagia is not black and white.

There is a vast gray area regarding tolerance of foods and liquids.

For example, after visiting an imaging center, you may think that the patient cannot drink thin liquids at all when, in fact, he may be able to manage with a chin tuck, verbal cues, or being careful not to wash foods down with liquids. He may simply be weak with a temporary swallowing problem and would benefit from exercises to improve his muscle coordination, strength and timing when swallowing.

Imaging center staff may not recommend that the patient follow up with a speech pathologist to address the need for swallowing therapy. They may not know to check the patient's position during the examination, or assess his risk with straw drinking or note where and how the fluids travel. They are not likely to provide barium-coated foods to determine what he can and cannot eat safely. The procedure is more likely to resemble an upper GI than a swallow test.

In my clinical opinion, you—the caregiver—should not leave without adequate information about how the patient manages both solids and liquids. If a VFSS (or MBSS) procedure is deemed to be the ideal test for the patient, I would advise that you schedule it through your local hospital radiology department as an outpatient procedure. The best and most comprehensive information is gathered through a team approach with the speech pathologist and the radiologist working together to recommend the safest patient-specific plan for your loved one's particular chewing or swallowing impairment.

CHOOSING A TEST

Speech pathologists have differing clinical perspectives regarding which test they prefer and often weigh factors when recommending a procedure. Most will agree that any test is better than no test.

Below are some considerations that may make one test preferable over another, but there may be other factors that are not listed. It is best to consult with your physician and speech pathologist when you are trying to decide which test is best.

VFSS or MBSS (Barium Test)
This procedure is beneficial if:
- There are concerns about esophageal problems such as stricture (a narrowing of the esophagus) generally caused by chronic gastroesophageal reflux disease— better known as "reflux." The physician can write an order for additional testing such as an upper GI to be performed directly after the initial swallowing test. This eliminates the need for a second appointment.
- To better determine function of the throat muscles.
- To assess for trace amounts of aspiration that could be missed on the FEES.
- The individual cannot tolerate having a scope placed in his nasal cavity for the course of the test.
- He is too confused to participate in a FEES evaluation.

FEES

This procedure is preferable if:
- Radiation exposure is a concern.
- The patient is obese. VFSS chair and instruments cannot accommodate obese patients easily and, sometimes, not at all.
- Fatigue is suspected as a factor in her tolerance of foods and liquids.
- If she has reduced mobility, such as confinement to the ICU, ventilator dependent, or she is in isolation due to an infection.
- She is unable to control her saliva.
- If she has dementia will not likely eat barium-coated foods.

Regardless of the test methods you choose, the information gathered will give you the most accurate picture of the patient's swallow function and provide you with functional information about how to manage his dysphagia.

CHAPTER 6

REFLUX DISEASE VERSUS FUNCTIONAL SWALLOWING DISORDERS

During my first few years working as an SLP, my role in managing swallowing disorders at the level of the esophagus was minor and was limited to carrying over any instructions from the treating physician. Indications that the problem might be related to a digestive issue meant that the patient was sent for a gastroenterology consult.

Currently, ASHA's Code of Ethics now lists the esophageal phase of swallowing as an area SLP's may offer guidance and management of symptoms, however this management is very limited and should be provided in collaboration with the physician. The SLP must have dysphagia evaluation and treatment experience and be qualified to study the patient's symptoms and to determine the source of the problem. Though the SLP does not "diagnose" problems of the esophagus, she records symptoms and suspected problems as a part of the initial evaluation and subsequent treatment reports and reports the information to the physician.

During the evaluation, the SLP will consider whether the dysphagia may be caused by the way the patient swallows (functional), or if the difficulty is moving foods through the throat to the stomach. She will question the patient about patterns that may occur, such as: Does he get the foods down and then experience burping and reflux after swallowing? Does he cough or vomit up foamy saliva? Does he experience nausea or vomiting with certain foods or under certain conditions? Are his symptoms worse at night? If so, the patient needs to see a doctor qualified to diagnose and treat these symptoms.

The gastroenterologist, ENT and your family physician are essential in managing diseases and disorders of the esophagus. The SLP's role is limited to isolating where the swallowing problem may occur (esophagus or other areas), and in making recommendations to help manage the symptoms. While the SLP may provide diet consistency recommendations or strategies to reduce reflux or to improve management of foods when certain structural changes have been diagnosed (such as an esophageal stricture or a web), esophageal problems should be diagnosed and managed by your physician.

Signs of esophageal problems should be immediately reported to, and assessed by, a gastroenterologist or an otolaryngologist (ENT) to determine the nature of the problem, and to rule out more serious conditions.

CHAPTER 7

TO TUBE OR NOT TO TUBE: END OF LIFE CARE

"Dad has had all those tests and he's still having trouble." There are times when, no matter what we try, the individual with dysphagia continues to have significant difficulty chewing and swallowing. In some cases, it is lack of compliance that is the problem. That is, he is either unwilling or unable to apply the techniques that have been recommended to reduce his choking and aspiration risks.

In the case of unwillingness, it is often because he dislikes the recommended food or liquid consistencies. In other instances, it is simply that he is unable to understand what he needs to do (such as tuck his chin to swallow). Those with severe cognitive deficits may be unable to remember and apply the steps needed to chew and swallow safely. In other cases, there may be extensive neurological damage from diseases such as stroke, Multiple Sclerosis or Parkinson's disease. Both of these diseases affect both physical and mental function.

A WORD ON FREQUENT COLD OR ALLERGY SYMPTOMS

I am always suspicious of an "asthma" diagnosis in an elderly patient who has never had asthma or breathing problems until the current problem arises. If your parent or spouse is experiencing chronic congestion, or has repeated bouts of bronchitis, it may be more than a seasonal problem, such as the congestion brought on by colds, influenza or allergies. These symptoms could be the result of chronic penetration or aspiration of foods and/or liquids into his lungs. Pay close attention to an increase in respiratory illnesses. What may seem like an allergy or a cold could be something more serious. If this sounds familiar, ask your physician to consider an objective swallow study.

FEEDING TUBES: END OF LIFE CONSIDERATIONS

Managing pain is universal in healthcare settings for the most part, but every person has a different notion about what defines "quality of life" and whether or not they want life sustaining and extending measures. It is easier on you and your loved ones if decisions about life-saving or life-extending measures such as cardiopulmonary resuscitation (CPR), breathing or feeding tubes are made prior to complete decline. If a person stops eating and she does not want a feeding tube, an Advanced Directive can give make the process easier for family and caregivers knowing that they are honoring her wishes. Encourage those in your care to fill out an Advanced Directive or to prepare a Living Will that tells caregivers and family what she would like them to do if she is unable to tell them directly.

Most physicians now have Advanced Directive forms that you can request during a routine visit, or—if your parent or spouse is hospitalized, or in a long-term care facility—ask the social worker where you can obtain this form.

While I do not endorse any particular organization, Caring Connections at www.caringinfo.org, a program of the National Hospice and Palliative Care Organization (NHPCO) offers advanced directive forms to individuals, by state, at no charge. There is a link on the right side of the website for "state specific" advanced directive forms. The forms can be printed (PDF) for personal use. The site and the forms are copyrighted. Any organization that wants to use Caring Connections forms for other than individual use must contact them at the number listed on their website for permission to mass distribute the forms.

SUMMARY

In conclusion, dysphagia is a swallowing disorder than can be mild or serious. Swallowing problems do not simply "go away" without treatment. If you, a spouse, parent or someone in your care experiences problems with chewing or swallowing, always, without exception, contact her physician to report the problem and seek guidance on how best to manage it.

Ask the physician for a speech therapy referral to determine the nature of the chewing or swallowing disorder, particularly if she is getting weaker, having more difficulty speaking clearly or has a history of stroke or other neurological diseases such as Parkinson's disease. Even if she is unable to directly participate in a therapy program, you, the caregiver may benefit from professional advice on how to manage her swallowing disorder or prevent decline. If she has difficulty maintaining weight or has a history of poor eating, consult a dietitian to learn ways to manage her nutrition.

Remember, you are not alone. In many cases, dysphagia can be managed with diet consistency changes and safety strategies. Millions of people are living with, and managing, dysphagia. You can manage it, too.

AUTHOR

S.G. Garbin is a nonfiction writer and speech pathologist, and a novelist with works of fiction and poetry published under the name Gabrielle Garbin. She lives in the Northeast with her husband and an Irish setter, Finn, better known as "the sweetest dog who ever lived."

Author Qualifications: I have been a practicing speech pathologist for seventeen years. I have performed hundreds of videofluoroscopic (barium and x-ray) swallow studies, treated numerous patients with dysphagia, and counseled their caregivers and families on how to help their patients and loved ones manage dysphagia.

I hope you found this book helpful in managing the swallowing problems of the elderly person in your care. To find my other books of fiction and poetry, or to read my writing blog, please visit:
https://www.smashwords.com/profile/view/GabrielleGarbin

You can also connect with me at:
Blog: www.gabriellegarbinblog.wordpress.com
Twitter: https://twitter.com/garbingabrielle
Facebook: https://www.facebook.com/gabrielle.garbin
Wattpad: http://www.wattpad.com/user/GabrielleGarbin
Pinterest: http://pinterest.com/gabriellegarbin
Linked In: www.linkedin.com/pub/gabrielle-garbin/6b/204/114/
Website: http://www.GabrielleGarbin.com

DISCLAIMER

What this book is: This book is written for you, the caregiver. Though it is not written for medical professionals who routinely work with dysphagia patients, it may be a resource guide for their patients, students, certified nursing assistants and home healthcare workers. The information provided inside this book comes from both my years of practice, from search engine results for the most current information using sites such as Wikipedia and Dysphagia.com. I have included links to YouTube videos to further the reader's understanding of how normal and disordered swallowing appears in a testing situation.

What this book is not: This book is not a substitute for medical, nutritional or legal advice, or the advice of the SLP you may be working with at present. You should consult your physician about any changes in medical status including difficulty talking, thinking clearly or chewing and/or swallowing foods. If you or someone you are caring for has a medical condition such as aspiration pneumonia, difficulty swallowing or is coughing or choking during meals, please contact his physician immediately.

Made in the USA
San Bernardino, CA
07 June 2015